FIT SPIRIT

BRYAN & STEPHANIE VIGNERY

Keep FIT SPIRIT by your bedside.

Let a devotional thought from God's Word be the first words you read and the last words you review today.

Copyright © 2020 by Bryan & Stephanie Vignery

Fit Spirit
By Bryan & Stephanie Vignery

ISBN-13: 978-1-7345640-2-0

All rights reserved. This book may not be reproduced in whole or in part in any form or format without permission in writing from the author, except for brief quotations in a review.

Bible quotations marked (NIV) are taken from THE HOLY BIBLE, NEW INTERNATIONAL VERSION®, NIV® Copyright © 1973, 1978, 1984, 2011 by Biblica, Inc.® Used by permission. All rights reserved worldwide.

Bible quotations marked (NKJV) are taken from the New King James Version®. Copyright © 1982 by Thomas Nelson. Used by permission. All rights reserved.

Bible quotations marked (NLT) are taken from Holy Bible, New Living Translation, copyright © 1996, 2004, 2015 by Tyndale House Foundation. Used by permission of Tyndale House Publishers Inc., Carol Stream, Illinois 60188. All rights reserved.

Bible quotation marked (NASB) is taken from the NEW AMERICAN STANDARD BIBLE®, Copyright © 1960, 1962, 1963, 1968, 1971, 1972, 1973, 1975, 1977, 1995 by The Lockman Foundation. Used by permission.

DAY ONE

Fear seems to be common in today's culture. People are discouraged by the fear in their lives when they allow it to control them. God said He would uphold us with His righteous right hand, and being held by Jesus doesn't leave any room for fear. Embrace the truth that He will be with you.

"For I am the LORD your God,
who upholds your right hand,
Who says to you,
'Do not fear, I will help you.'"

(Isaiah 41:13 NASB)

DAY TWO

With Jesus' strength, our limitations become unlimited. Not that Jesus will give us superpowers to do things that are physically impossible, but He will do the supernatural for those who press into Him.

I can do all things through Christ
who strengthens me.

(Philippians 4:13 NKJV)

FIT SPIRIT

DAY 2

DAY THREE

In today's culture, the idea of hope and a future can seem daunting. But, you have been created for a purpose, and driving that purpose is a plan that God has strategically designed for you. Allow His protection and plan to drive your purpose and desires.

"For I know the plans I have for you," declares the LORD, "plans to prosper you and not to harm you, plans to give you hope and a future."

(Jeremiah 29:11 NIV)

DAY FOUR

Trust can be a difficult thing. Many of us have seen from our upbringing, relationships, and other areas of life that trust can easily be broken. If we look to establish a trusting heart from our earthly relationships, we will be disappointed. But if we look to the Lord and submit our plans to Him, we will see our trust for others increase.

Trust in the LORD with all your heart
and lean not on your own understanding;
in all your ways submit to him,
and he will make your paths straight.

(Proverbs 3:5–6 NIV)

FIT SPIRIT

DAY 4

DAY FIVE

Here is a simple truth; garbage in, garbage out. We pay the price in some fashion for what we allow in our lives. God desires to have our heart, and when He has it, He will provide the abundance needed to serve Him and others effectively.

A good man out of the good treasure of his heart brings forth good; and an evil man out of the evil treasure of his heart brings forth evil. For out of the abundance of the heart his mouth speaks.

(Luke 6:45 NKJV)

FIT SPIRIT

DAY SIX

Hiding can be fun when it's played as a game with your children. Hiding as an attempt to keep God in the dark sets us up for defeat. Knowing that God knows everything and doesn't desire to shame you can be an understanding of freedom!

But when you pray, go into your room,
close the door and pray to your Father,
who is unseen. Then your Father, who sees
what is done in secret, will reward you.

(Matthew 6:6 NIV)

FIT SPIRIT

DAY SEVEN

Overflow with confident hope? Sign me up! It is only through the power of the Holy Spirit that we can experience true hope, joy, and peace. It is a free gift to all who choose.

"I pray that God, the source of hope, will fill you completely with joy and peace because you trust in him. Then you will overflow with confident hope through the power of the Holy Spirit."

(Romans 15:13 NLT)

DAY EIGHT

Sin is a choice that can be embraced or rejected. Therefore, we do not have to be controlled by the sin in our life. We have a choice, daily, to seek more of the Holy Spirit and live in the fullness of Christ within us.

But you are not controlled by your sinful nature. You are controlled by the Spirit if you have the Spirit of God living in you. (And remember that those who do not have the Spirit of Christ living in them do not belong to him at all.) And Christ lives within you, so even though your body will die because of sin, the Spirit gives you life because you have been made right with God.

(Romans 8:9-10 NLT)

FIT SPIRIT

DAY NINE

People change. Seasons change — the weather changes. Pretty much everything changes over time, except Jesus. He is the one and only real constant in a world where the norm is change. Rest in the assurance that Jesus will not be like those that disappoint you in life. He will be the same, always.

Jesus Christ is the same
yesterday, today, and forever.

(Hebrews 13:8 NKJV)

FIT SPIRIT

DAY 9

DAY TEN

Troubled hearts are a product of the disappointments of this world. True peace is from the Lord and will sustain even when the world disappoints.

"Peace I leave with you, My peace I give to
you; not as the world gives do I give to you.
Let not your heart be troubled,
neither let it be afraid."

(John 14:27 NKJV)

FIT SPIRIT

DAY ELEVEN

We all have to overcome struggles in our lives. Although we may face some struggles that seem insurmountable, there is no struggle that cannot be conquered by God. So, remember, you are an overcomer because He overcame the world!

"I have told you these things, so that in me you may have peace. In this world you will have trouble. But take heart! I have overcome the world."

(John 16:33 NIV)

DAY TWELVE

It has always amazed me that we can easily light up the night with something as small as a match. But no matter how hard we try, we cannot invade the light with a small piece of darkness. Light is powerful, and we can walk in it every day! Allowing Jesus to be the light of our work will surely drive out the darkness.

Then Jesus spoke to them again, saying, "I am the light of the world. He who follows Me shall not walk in darkness, but have the light of life."

(John 8:12 NKJV)

FIT SPIRIT

DAY THIRTEEN

As a parent, I cannot fathom the thought of giving up one of my children. The fact of the matter is, the true Father gave up His Son for us. What a powerful example of Love sacrificed for others.

For God so loved the world that He gave His only begotten Son, that whoever believes in Him should not perish but have everlasting life.

(John 3:16 NKJV)

FIT SPIRIT

DAY 13

DAY FOURTEEN

Fear is a spirit. God gives us power, love, and a sound mind. The enemy wants to take away your power, love, and the soundness of your mind. Don't give in to the spirit of fear, but cast it out in the name of Jesus!

For God has not given us a spirit of fear,
but of power and of love
and of a sound mind.

(2 Timothy 1:7 NKJV)

FIT SPIRIT

DAY 14

DAY FIFTEEN

It makes God happy when we seek Him first, above everything else.

And it is impossible to please God without faith. Anyone who wants to come to him must believe that God exists and that he rewards those who sincerely seek him.

(Hebrews 11:6 NLT)

FIT SPIRIT

DAY SIXTEEN

God's got this! He sees the future; we don't. We have to trust and know that God wants the best for us and that no matter what comes our way, He will see us through it.

Faith shows the reality
of what we hope for;
it is the evidence of things we cannot see.

(Hebrews 11:1 NLT)

FIT SPIRIT

DAY SEVENTEEN

God is our ultimate strength, no matter what. We need not worry. God lifts us up in our deepest valleys, and no matter what, He will keep us strong, even our weakest moments, because God is strong.

But those who trust in the LORD
will find new strength.
They will soar high on wings like eagles.
They will run and not grow weary.
They will walk and not faint.

(Isaiah 40:31 NLT)

FIT SPIRIT

DAY EIGHTEEN

God is standing right here with open arms, saying, "I am here to take your burdens upon Myself. I never said life would be easy. I did say that I would be with you and see you through to the end. I will never leave. I will not abandon you."

"Come to me, all you who are weary and burdened, and I will give you rest. Take my yoke upon you and learn from me, for I am gentle and humble in heart, and you will find rest for your souls. For my yoke is easy and my burden is light."

(Matthew 11:28–30 NIV)

FIT SPIRIT

DAY NINETEEN

The greatest commandment is to love the One who loves you most, with every part of your being. The next is to put your own love into action for the benefit of others.

So he answered and said, "'You shall love the LORD your God with all your heart, with all your soul, with all your strength, and with all your mind,' and 'your neighbor as yourself.'"

(Luke 10:27 NKJV)

FIT SPIRIT

DAY TWENTY

It's true that we cannot control what we cannot control. But when we worry about it, we show a lack of faith in God. There is no need to worry. God is completely in control of your circumstances. He's got you, so He's got this!

Therefore do not worry about tomorrow, for tomorrow will worry about itself. Each day has enough trouble of its own.

(Matthew 6:34 NIV)

FIT SPIRIT

DAY TWENTY-ONE

You never have to doubt the truth of God when you follow the word of God. God is the truth, and by knowing Him, you can find hope and freedom for every circumstance in your life.

To the Jews who had believed him, Jesus said, "If you hold to my teaching, you are really my disciples. Then you will know the truth, and the truth will set you free."

(John 8:31–32 NIV)

DAY TWENTY-TWO

It doesn't often seem that God is quick to act, but in my experience, I've found that His timing is always perfect. He has never failed me. No matter what, evil will never defeat good. God has defeated Satan; always has and always will.

Be still in the presence of the LORD,
and wait patiently for him to act.
Don't worry about evil people who prosper
or fret about their wicked schemes.

(Psalm 37:7 NLT)

DAY TWENTY-THREE

The enemy is on the prowl, but God has given us power. Bind Satan in the name of Jesus and resist his evil schemes. He will never have power over you nor harm you. This is a great promise of God that provides great security.

Submit yourselves, then, to God.
Resist the devil, and he will flee from you.

(James 4:7 NIV)

DAY TWENTY-FOUR

God has plans and purposes for each one of us. It's up to us to fulfill the purposes to which He has called us. Through Jesus, He has given us the ultimate example—to show us how to put His plans for us into action!

And we know that all things work together for good to those who love God, to those who are the called according to His purpose.

(Romans 8:28 NKJV)

FIT SPIRIT

DAY TWENTY-FIVE

Just as a parent wants to bless their child with wonderful things, God's blessings far exceed our imagination! And it's okay to ask for God's blessings in our life. He wants to bless us, but sometimes, He is waiting for us to come to Him.

And Jabez called on the God of Israel saying, "Oh, that You would bless me indeed, and enlarge my territory, that Your hand would be with me, and that You would keep me from evil, that I may not cause pain!" So God granted him what he requested.

(1 Chronicles 4:10 NKJV)

FIT SPIRIT

DAY TWENTY-SIX

God is always here to lift us up and carry our burdens, whether heavy or light. He never takes our burdens lightly. What burdens do you need to give to the Lord today?

Give your burdens to the LORD,
and he will take care of you.
He will not permit the godly to slip and fall.

(Psalm 55:22 NLT)

FIT SPIRIT

DAY TWENTY-SEVEN

God gives us the desires of our hearts for a reason. No matter what, when we leave everything in His hands, He will make sure it comes to fruition. Trust is developed through faith in the Lord and will create peace and security in your life.

Commit your way to the LORD,
Trust also in Him,
And He shall bring it to pass.

(Psalm 37:5 NKJV)

FIT SPIRIT

DAY TWENTY-EIGHT

We cannot endure the toughest challenges in our own strength, with our own abilities. When we allow God to be the Lord of our lives, He becomes the source of our strength and courage through all of the challenges we face.

"Be strong and courageous, because you will lead these people to inherit the land I swore to their ancestors to give them."

* * *

"Have I not commanded you? Be strong and courageous. Do not be afraid; do not be discouraged, for the LORD your God will be with you wherever you go."

(Joshua 1:6, 9 NIV)

FIT SPIRIT

DAY TWENTY-NINE

FIT SPIRIT

To move forward in all God has for us, we have to forget what is behind us. Until we do, we are holding ourselves back.

"Not that I have already obtained all this, or have already arrived at my goal, but I press on to take hold of that for which Christ Jesus took hold of me. Brothers and sisters, I do not consider myself yet to have taken hold of it. But one thing I do: Forgetting what is behind and straining toward what is ahead, I press on toward the goal to win the prize for which God has called me heavenward in Christ Jesus."

(Philippians 3:12–14 NIV)

FIT SPIRIT

DAY THIRTY

Seek God first, and no less than this.

Seek the Kingdom of God above all else,
and live righteously, and he will give you
everything you need.

(Matthew 6:33 NLT)

FIT SPIRIT

DAY THIRTY-ONE

Give thanks to God in everything. When He starts something in you, He will finish it. No matter what the outcome, it will be God who receives the glory for it all.

Consider it pure joy, my brothers and sisters, whenever you face trials of many kinds, because you know that the testing of your faith produces perseverance. Let perseverance finish its work so that you may be mature and complete,
not lacking anything.

(James 1:2–4 NIV)

FIT SPIRIT

www.ingramcontent.com/pod-product-compliance
Lightning Source LLC
Chambersburg PA
CBHW081126080526
44587CB00021B/3759